A Day in The Life Of Russell Sprout

A sprout is for life, not just for Christmas

I.M. Mayes

A Day in The Life of Russell Sprout

Copyright © *I.M. Mayes*, 2025

All Rights Reserved

This book is subject to the condition that no part of this book is to be reproduced, transmitted in any form or means; electronic or mechanical, stored in a retrieval system, photocopied, recorded, scanned, or otherwise. Any of these actions require the proper written permission of the author.

Contents

Chapter 1 – The Introduction 5

Chapter 2 – A Fresh New Day 17

Chapter 3 – Disruption 23

Chapter 4 – Revealing their Dreams and Plans for The Future 32

Chapter 5 – Welcoming the New Pupils 45

NHS Guidelines 5 a Day 55

Chapter 1 – The Introduction

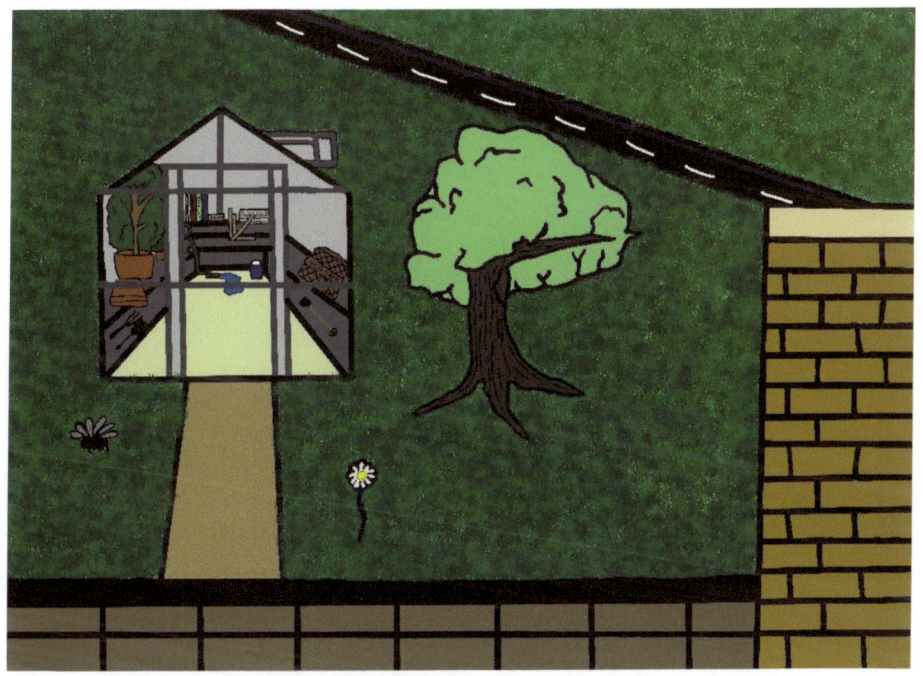

"I was lucky to be born into a vast and beautiful landscape in late spring—with fields and fertile farmland stretching as far as the eye could see. The crisp, fresh air and an abundance of sunshine made it the perfect setting for me to grow and thrive. Honestly, who could have asked for anything more beautiful than this? My name is Russell, Russell Sprout, and this is my story."

And so, Russell's story began—not in a classroom or a playground, but on a quiet patch of fertile earth, lovingly cared for by the one he called Father.

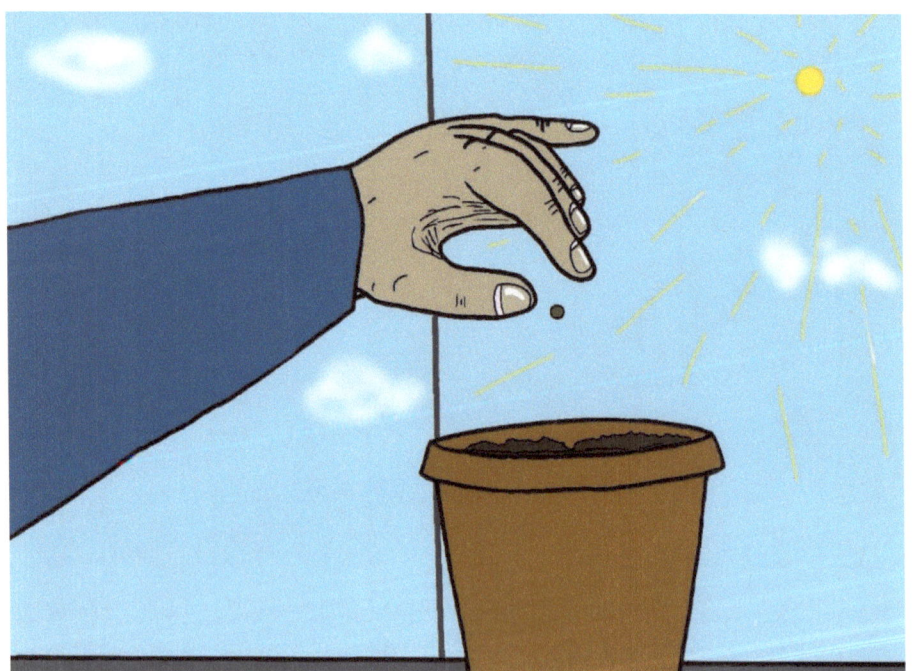

Russell Sprout had been planted with care, given the best soil, and raised beneath clear skies and golden sun. His father—his human father—tended to him every day, making sure he had everything he needed to grow strong and healthy.

Father always spoke to him as he grew. He would often say, "One day, you will be something special. You can be anything you want to be if you put your mind to it."

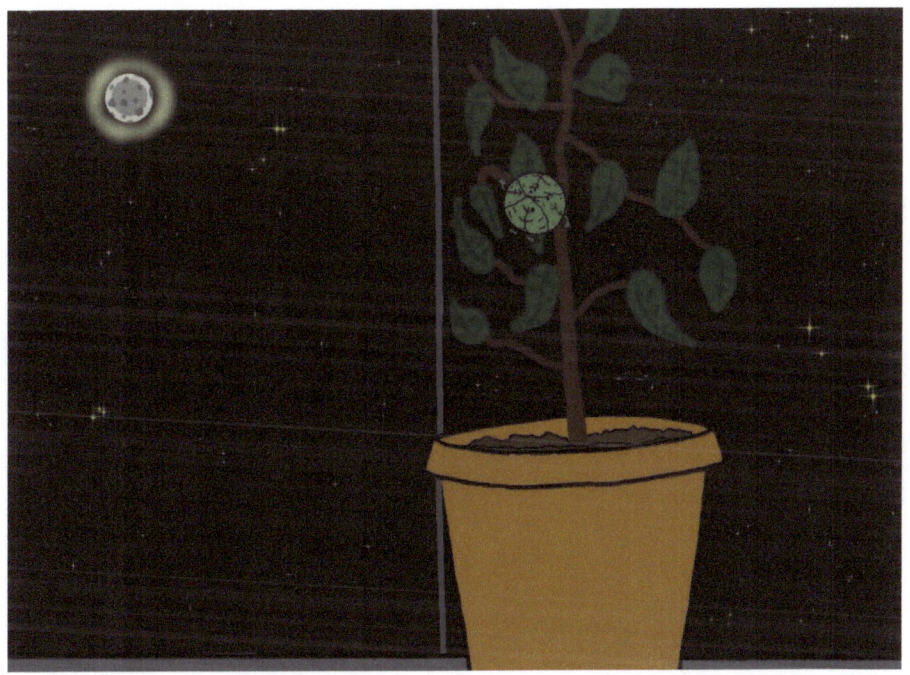

After a good day with plenty of sunshine, the night began to fall. The moon rose into the night sky, and Russell could feel himself growing bigger.

Half asleep and still hanging on from his branch, Father woke him up. "Come on, Russell Sprout, it is time for you to go to school."

Russell replied, "School? What School, Father?"

And just as he asked, there was a tapping on the windowpane. A delivery man handed him a parcel.

"Here we are Russell, I have imported your headteacher from the USA— there was no stock at the local supermarket."

"Confused and bewildered, I hung from the branch, staring as Father carefully opened the parcel with his scissors. He peeled back the packaging, and a long, green character popped her head out of the box."

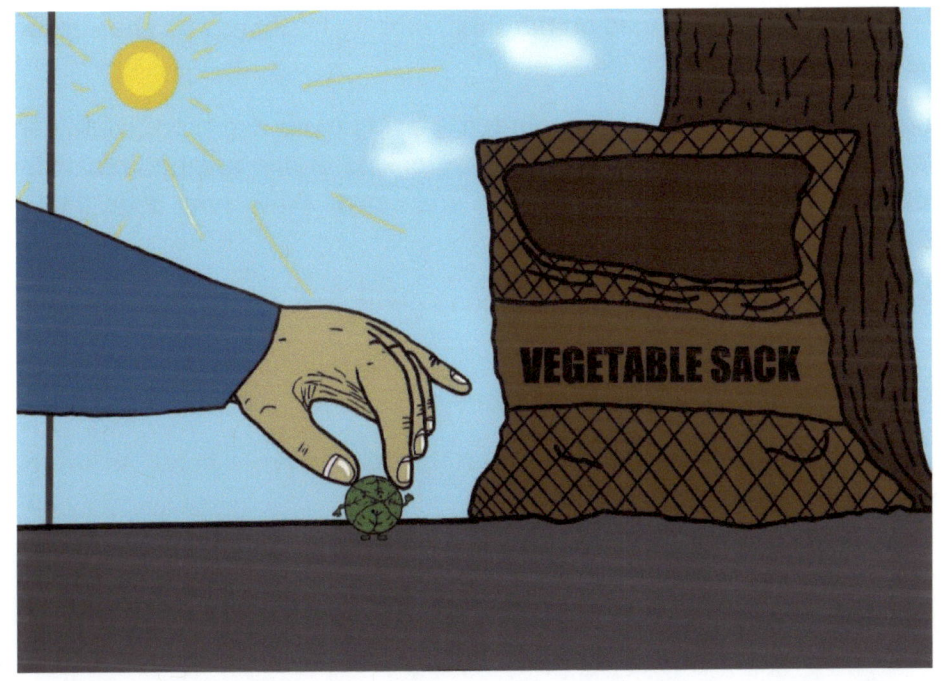

"With a quick snip, Father clipped me from the branch, gently picked me up, and placed me on the shelf."

"There you go, Russell. It is time for you to meet your new headmistress, Miss Scallion." Puzzled Russell looked at her with his mouth wide open as he did not know what to say.

Miss Scallion leapt from the box and landed on the shelf, rubbing her hands as she strolled across the shelf while calling, "Where are the rest of my pupils?"

Father began snipping at other plants from his garden, placing more and more characters beside me and Miss Scallion. Soon, the shelf was full of curious faces, looking at one another in wonder. Without saying goodbye, Father quietly left the building. He opened and closed the school door, then walked down the garden path to his house.

Miss Scallion blew a whistle and called out, "Everybody get in line. Pupils, it is the time we all learn one another's names".

Then everybody scuttled around and got in the line and in position.

First in the line was Russell. Miss Scallion moved her glasses down her nose, as she bent down, looked directly at him "And who are you, my dear?" she asked.

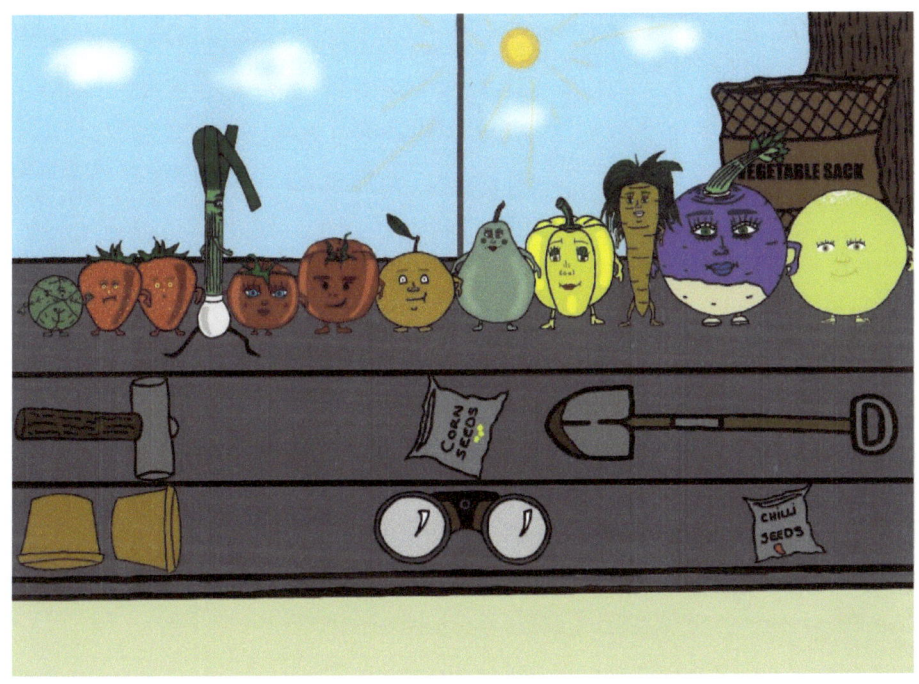

Russell replied, "I am Russell Sprout, Miss." He waved and she walked further down the line. Miss Scallion came to the pupils who were second in the line, they look related, Russell pondered. Russell looked on and further down the line.

Miss Scallion asked, "And what are your names?" The two characters sang in unison, "Terry and Jenny, the berries miss, we are strawberries." Miss Scallion asked them another question, "are you related at all?" They both looked at one another and said, "Yes, miss, we are brother and sister. We grew up on the same plant together."

"How lovely!" she said, walking further down the line to the fourth pupil.

"You look very sweet poppit, and who are you?" The little cherry tomato felt a little shy, and her face turned redder while replying, "My name is Cherie Tomato, she giggled and carried on saying, this is my friend Tommy Tomato." Miss Scallion greeted Tommy, who was next in the line.

Walking further, she came across the next pupil. "Hello, my dear! Who are you?"

"Hello, Miss, I am Clem." Miss Scallion, out of curiosity, asked, "Clem, what kind of name is that?"

"It's short for Clementine, Miss," she replied. Miss Scallion was taken aback a little and said, "Your friends can call you this, but I only address pupils by their full names, so I will call you Clementine." Clementine responded, "Okay, Miss," as Miss Scallion moved on to the next pupil.

"Hello, name, please?" Miss Scallion asked. "I am Cher the pear. Nice to meet you." Miss Scallion smiled at Cher. And responded, "The pleasure is all mine" as she walked further down the line.

"My goodness, aren't you sweet? And what is your name?" Miss Scallion asked the next pupil.

"Thank you. Miss, my name is Belle Pepper."

Miss Scallion replied, "Nice to meet you, sweet pepper!"

Continuing walking down the line. Only three more pupils to go.

She asked, "And what is your name, please?"

"Hello, Miss, I am Julienne the carrot." Miss Scallion added, "Oh, isn't that a fancy name?"

Julienne replied, "Thank you, I am happy you like my name." Miss Scallion had a smile on her face and replied, "Well, it's a wonderful name," while walking further down the line.

Miss Scallion asked the next one in the line, "Hello! And your name.? What is your name, my dear?"

"Tina, Miss. Tina turnip." Miss Scallion, as she walked further, said: "Lovely to meet you, Tina Turnip."

Finally, it was the last pupil to be seen.

Without even asking, an excited pupil blasted her name out, "I am Helen Melon, Miss." Miss Scallion smiled while looking at Helen and replied: "And I am Miss Scallion. Class, welcome to Green House Elementary. Pupils, if you ever have any problems while you are here— if there is anything you would like to ask or need to know—then please remember: I am your new headmistress. Feel free to come and see me in my office. I would also like to say that you all seem lovely pupils, and I hope you enjoy your time here." With that, Miss Scallion suddenly blew her whistle to get everyone's attention.

"Okay, now that we all know each other's names, you are entitled to a fifteen-minute break. Go and explore your new school, and come back to me when you hear the whistle. Once your break is over, I will introduce you to your teachers. Now go, pupils— go!" she said, blowing the whistle once again.

All the pupils started scattering around with excitement, running around and exploring their new school. The greenhouse was filled with the sound of laughter and curiosity as Miss Scallion went to her office to do some paperwork.

Russell and his new friends explored the whole school. They found the library, Miss Scallion's office and their dormitory (where they will all sleep and spend the night), which was just a vegetable sack.

Russell and his friends found many items dotted around the school, from packets of seeds, plant pots, scissors and binoculars. Tools and other gardening equipment.

Russell and his friends noticed there were other shelves too below them and they found a garden hose that they could slide down to get to lower levels or the floor if they ever needed to. But being on the top shelf was great to get a full view of the school and garden.

Russell and his friends were getting to know one another—playing games and joking around. They were all in hysterics after a joke Tina turnip had told, when an almighty screech from Miss Scallion's whistle filled the school. Startled, they looked up to see Miss Scallion standing in her office, which overlooked everything, blowing the whistle with firm determination.

Miss Scallion shouted, "Fifteen minutes break is over!" as she climbed down the wooden garden canes that served as her peculiar staircase to the office. She carefully made her way down the canes and onto the top shelf below. The pupils all gathered around her and waited for further instruction.

Miss Scallion told the pupils: "Because the sun has set, and it has been an exciting day for you all, it is now becoming late and dark outside. I have decided to let the teachers plan for their lessons tomorrow, so I will introduce you to them tomorrow morning. However, I would like you to meet our lovely and sweet Mrs Granny Smith, who will take you to your resting place— the dormitory."

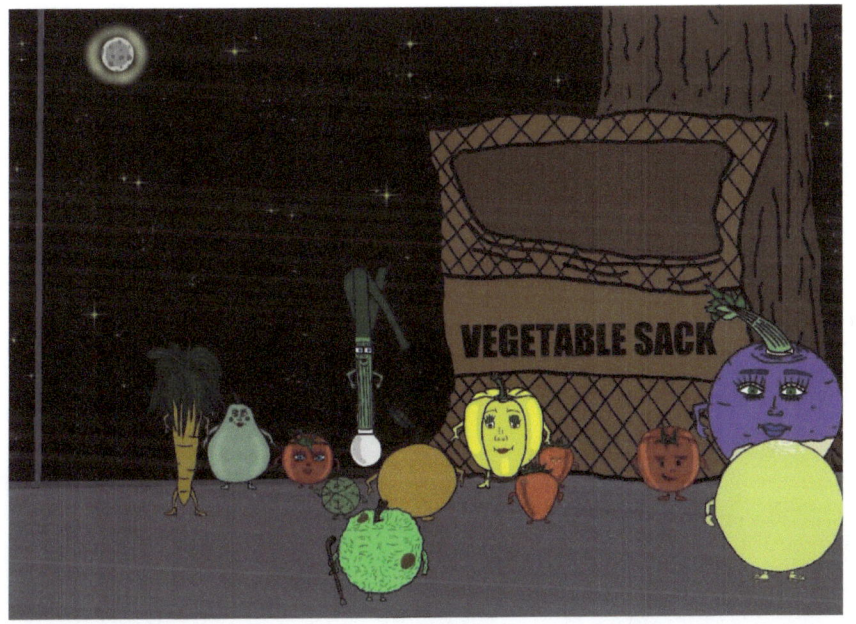

Just then, Mrs Granny Smith appeared quietly from behind the pupils as they were listening to Miss Scallion.

"Hello, children. Please come with me," she said kindly. The pupils followed Mrs Granny Smith in a slow but orderly fashion toward the vegetable sack. As they walked, Russell asked, "Why do you walk with a stick?"

Mrs Granny Smith let out a gentle laugh and replied, "When you are as old as me, dear, you start to go past your sell-by date. I am not as fresh or as young as I used to be, so I need a stick to help me get around."

As the moon hung in the night sky, Mrs Granny Smith turned to the children and said, "Get some rest, as it will be an even longer, busier day tomorrow with all your lessons."

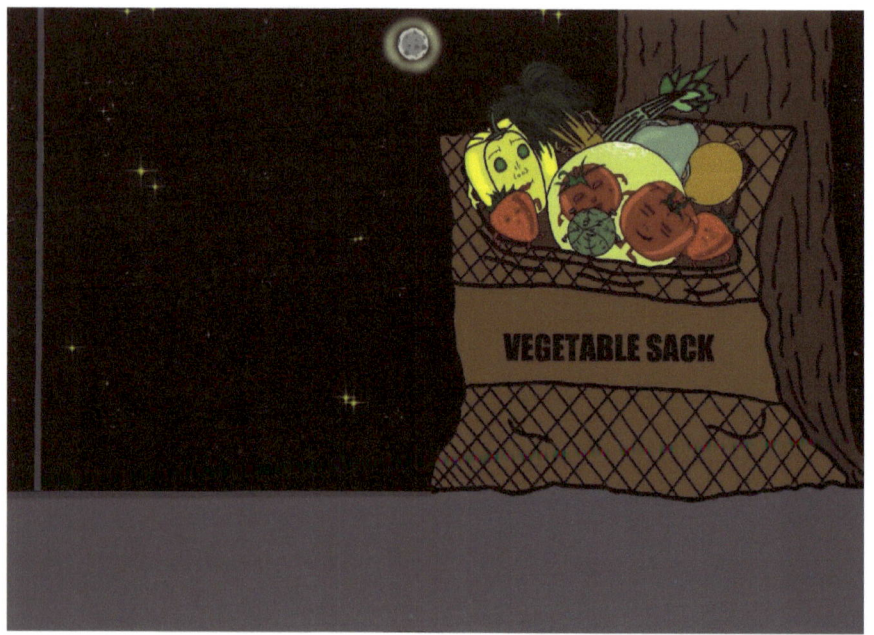

The fruit and vegetables, one by one, jumped into the vegetable sack and rested their eyes, ready for the day ahead.

Chapter 2 – A Fresh New Day

It was morning, and a fresh new day had begun. Sunlight shone brightly through the glass panes of the school, and the UV rays hit Russell, which energised him, leaving him rejuvenated and in a great mood. All the fruit and vegetables began to stir as Russell jumped out of the vegetable sack and onto the shelf. The other vegetables climbed out of the sack as well, and soon, everyone was talking and getting to know one another.

When Miss Scallion's whistle blew, she called out, "Come on, children, rise and shine as your first lesson is about to commence."

Russell and the rest of the class rushed to Miss Scallion. "The first lesson today will be Geography, and I will be teaching you this lesson. First and foremost, please collect your journals and pens. What I would like you all to do is go around the school and take in your surroundings and write or draw about the scenery from every windowpane. And just admire the beautiful area in which this fantastic school resides."

The pupils took their journals and pens and rushed off to different windowpanes, taking notes and drawing certain parts of the outside world. Russell found a window and pressed his face so hard into it to gaze at the beautiful natural world. He could not believe how perfect it was. Miss Scallion blew her whistle, and everyone returned to her. After a lot of excitement and discussion, the class showed each other's work to one another.

Miss Scallion told the class, "Come along, children. I have to take you to your next lesson; I need to introduce you to your new teachers", as she took large strides in a rush along the shelf with the fruit and vegetables following her.

Miss Scallion introduced the next class and teachers, "Your next lesson will be a gym class, and this will be taught by Mr Edward Potato. I would like to introduce you all to him and his wonderful wife, Jackie Potato. They are a lovely couple, and Jackie Potato will also be teaching art class today.."

Edward Potato and Jackie Potato appeared and greeted the pupils with a warm welcome. "Hello, pupils, today we are going to do some physical activity. Why is exercise important?" Edward asked the class.

Belle Pepper called out, "Is it to extend our lives?"

Mr Edward Potato called out to Belle Pepper, "Well, yes, it is for that reason. It does make us healthier just as it would a human. But please, Belle, when asked a question, don't just shout out. Please raise your hand if you have an answer."

Belle apologised, "Sorry, sir," after being told off.

Jackie Potato continued the conversation, "We, as fruits and vegetables, have a short shelf life; our days are shorter than human days. So now, it's time for your fifteen-minute break. Have fun and be safe, and after your break it's gym class with my husband, Edward."

Miss Scallion blew her whistle, and everyone started running around, playing and having fun.

Helen Melon approaches Russell. "Hey, Russell, do you like this school?" she asked.

"Yes, Helen Melon, it's a nice, fun place, and we get to learn, do you?" he asked.

"Yes, I think it is fabulous. We all feel really safe here," she replied while dashing away with Tina Turnip.

The two strawberries came and sat next to Russell Terry and Jenny said, "Hi Russell, how is your day going?" Before Russell could answer, Jenny said, "Oh, be quiet, brother. You think you're so special that Russell would want to speak to you? You think you're better than everyone else?"

Russell replied, "No, he doesn't. What's wrong with being kind to one another?" Terry walked off in a sulk.

Russell said to Jenny, "I thought you both are related. Why do you treat your brother like that?"

Jenny said, "Yes, we are, but he thinks he is better than everyone. Always Mr popular, and he is confident, I just don't like him."

"But, he's your brother," said Russell, and he was shocked to hear such animosity; he figured out that she was just jealous of him. But why so spiteful, he thought, clearly, as time had passed on, that jealousy had turned to envy and now hate. Russell decided to walk away from Jenny as he only liked to be around positive fruits and vegetables, and he felt Jenny seems to be someone you cannot trust, she clearly lies and makes things up just for sympathy and attention. It turned out she was not so sweet after all. Russell really liked

Terry. He doesn't say anything negative to others and is a positive chap. He guessed that Jenny never wanted her brother to shine or outgrow her.

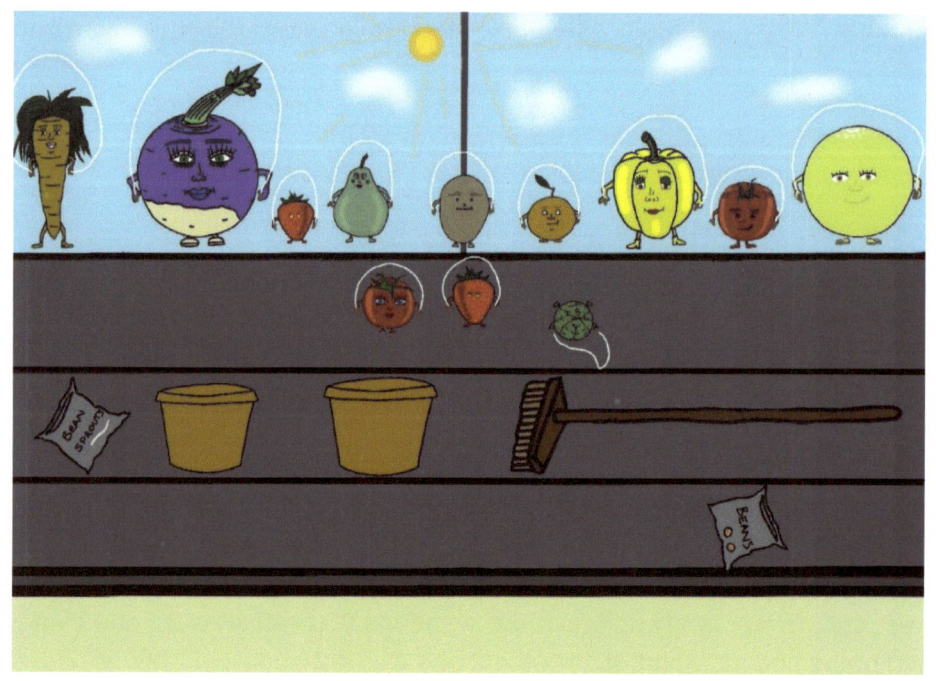

Miss Scallion blew her whistle to get everyone to gather up for gym class. Mr Edward Potato started by asking the pupils to "drop and give me twenty" as all the fruits and vegetables dropped to the floor and started doing push-ups. It went from push-ups to skip rope, and in no time,, all the fruit and vegetables were becoming exhausted. When Mr Edward Potato said, "Well done class! The majority of you really pushed yourselves hard there, and that was a great gym class. You should give yourselves a pat on the back."

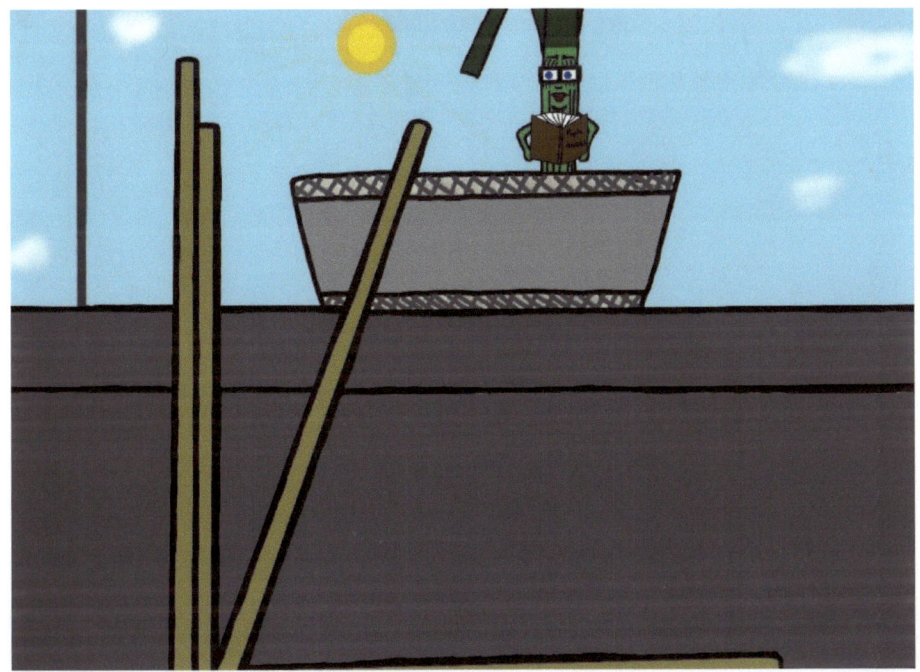

Miss Scallion walked back to her office to do paperwork, but she did notice Jenny Berry was not trying as hard as the rest at gym class.

The sun started to set, and everyone was beginning to yawn, which indicated it was time for bed. Mrs Jackie Potato called on the class, "It is getting late now, pupils. It is time for your rest. Can you please make your way to the dormitory in an orderly fashion.."

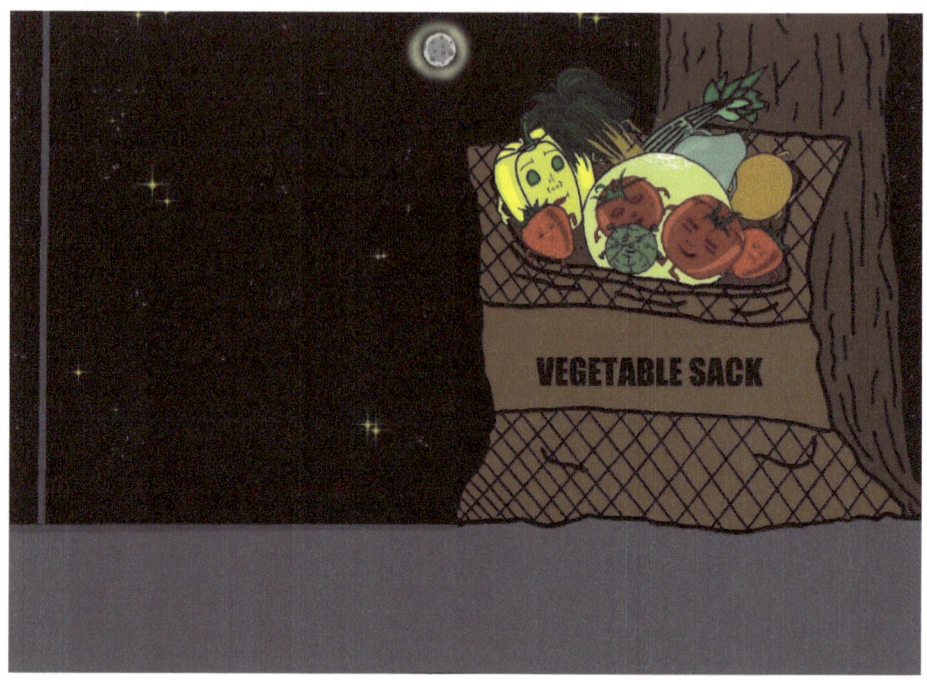

The fruits and vegetables made their way to the dormitory in a single file and jumped in their vegetable sack. They closed their eyes to see what the next day was going to bring.

Chapter 3 – Disruption

As night falls and the moon is back above Greenhouse Elementary, the fruits and vegetables are in a deep sleep, dreaming about their future, where or what they would like to be, before their best-before-date expires.

When suddenly and out of nowhere, an almighty crashing noise occurred, bang, bang, bang, wallop, bang, bang, bang.

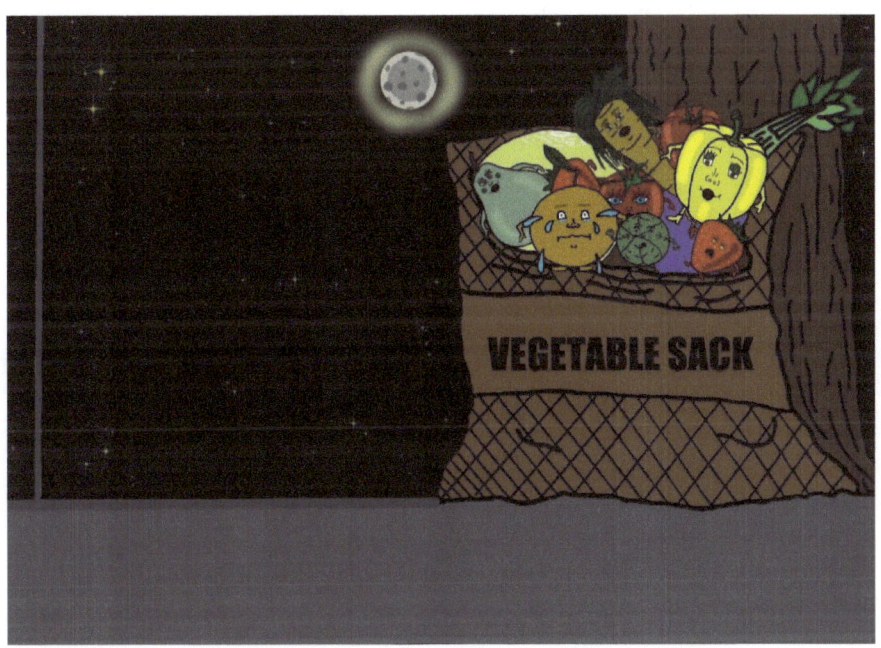

A screaming Clementine was crying in the bed "I don't like it, make it stop" as she cried and cried. Russell tried to make her feel better and didn't want her to worry. "Please, Clem, don't cry," he said. But Clementine would not stop crying.

Miss Scallion, Mr potato and Granny Smith came to the dormitory and called out, "What's all this commotion? What is that racket?" they asked. The noise was coming from outside, but it was too dark to see anything.

Miss Scallion tried to reassure the pupils to get some rest even though everyone was on the edge and the noises continued to go on. "Please, class, try to sleep. We will investigate this in the morning." The noises carried on throughout the night, and hardly anyone got any sleep.

Crash, bang, bang, wallop, crash, bang, bang, wallop, crash, bang, bang, wallop, crash, bang.

As the morning sun lights up the new day, everyone got out of the vegetable sack feeling a bit worse for wear with questions in their mind about the banging last night.

When an almighty scream bellowed and filled the greenhouse with more noise. Julienne, the carrot, pointed in the direction of the scream and started to rush towards it. The rest of the fruits and vegetables scuttled behind her. It was then that they all realised that it was Miss Scallion as she was looking out of the window.

A worried Cher, the pear asked her, "Miss Scallion, are you okay?"

"Oh, my goodness", she shouted.

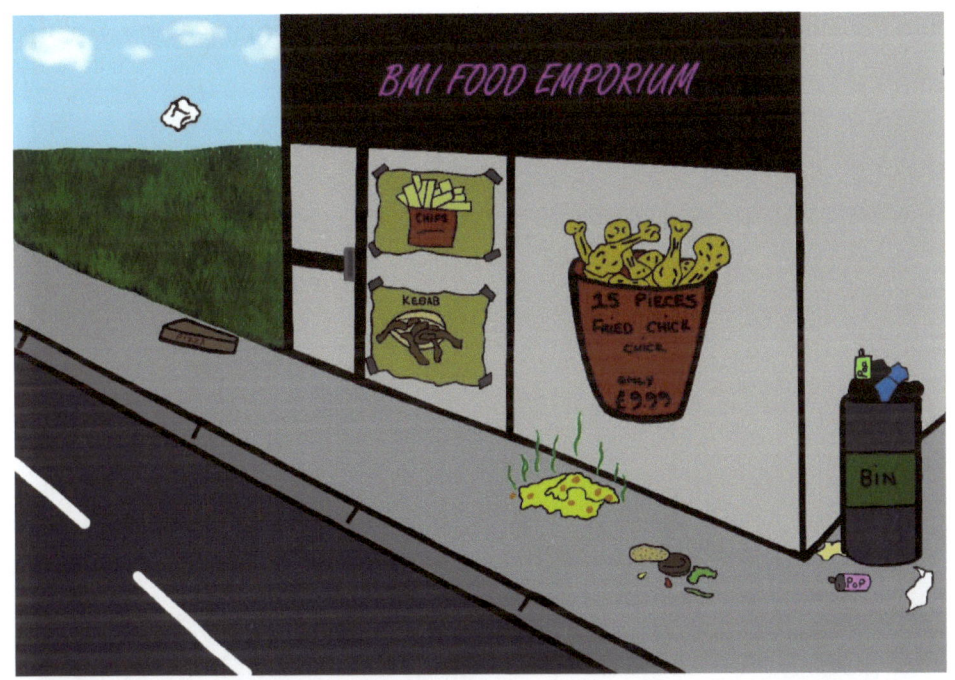

The whole class looked out of the window and noticed a new building had appeared nearby. There were noises, more humans and vehicles, and everything seemed much busier and louder. They watched on in terror as the natural environment that they grew to love so much was now being littered by some of the less-caring humans. They gained some hope when they saw other humans who must care about the natural environment as they placed their rubbish in the bin. But then even more humans arrived, and they just threw rubbish straight onto the streets, and some of them where piling more rubbish on a bin that was already full and then they would leave.

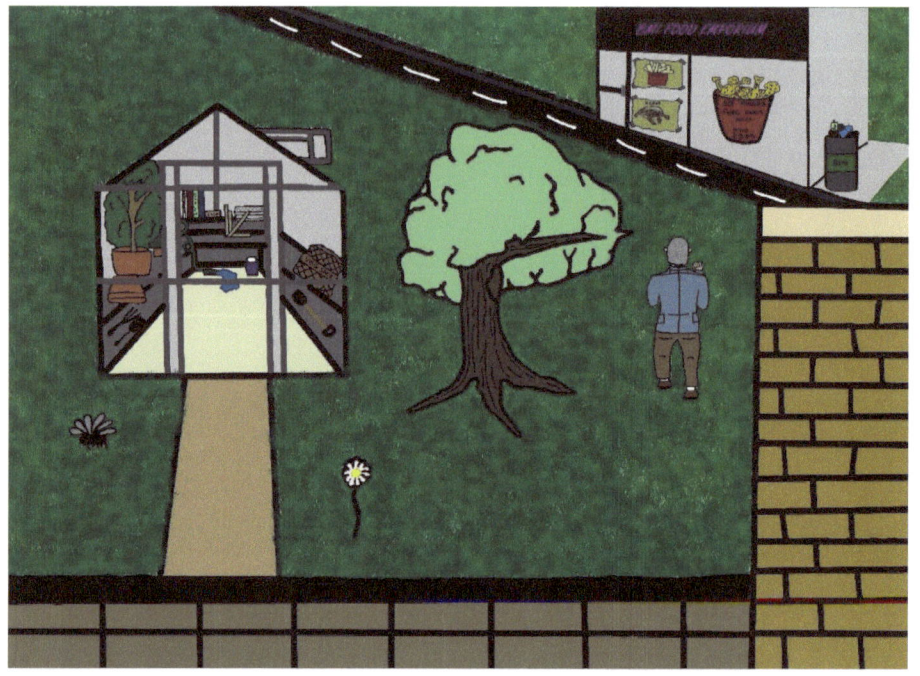

An angry father came out of his house and was shouting while raising his fist in the air. The fruits and vegetables could not hear what he was shouting about but it was evident he was not happy with the new building that appeared overnight.

A broken and upset Miss Scallion shed a few tears, and with a gentle, broken voice, she told the class, "Pupils, I am heartbroken today. I would like to go to my office to take a little time for myself." The other teachers arrived, and they could see how in despair the headmistress was. Edward and Jackie Potato, Granny Smith and a brand-new teacher revealed themselves and stood next to the other teachers. Edward escorted Miss Scallion to her office while Jackie and Granny Smith introduced the new teacher.

Granny Smith told the class, "Right. Pupils, last night and today, have struck us all hard. Things have changed around here now; I must enforce some school rules that must always be adhered to. Although you have never been outside our school and into the garden, we were going to take you outside on a school trip. However, we need to be more vigilant as we don't know of any hidden dangers that all these changes may bring. I would like to nominate a pupil to overlook and watch what is going on outside. This pupil can use the binoculars on the other shelf and keep an eye out, and their job is to report anything back to any teacher at once if they see anything or any dangers that may lurk. Let me have a think on who I will pick."

Jackie Potato then adds, "Today, lessons and the day will be cut shorter than usual; this will allow you all to have a little fun as the school trip is cancelled and in spite of recent events as we need to keep the mood in here positive and happy." When an argument broke out amongst the pupils.

Jenny Strawberry rolled her eyes and said in a very childish, snarly way, "Oh, why does everything have to be positive around here."

Terry Strawberry argued with Jenny, "Be quiet, Jenny."

Jenny Strawberry said so nastily, "No, Terry, I don't like positivity. I much prefer to be awkward and negative, and I don't like you."

"But why? Being negative drains everyone else, and you are my sister. Are you some kind of energy vampire?" He asked, and the whole class giggled except for Jenny, as she gave him a dirty look.

Mrs Jackie Potato snaps, "Enough, enough class! We want to keep it positive in here, and if Jenny doesn't like it, she can go to the headmistress's office to write lines as punishment."

Jenny gives a further snarl to Jackie, and Jackie tells her off "Just go, Jenny. Life is too short to put up with negative behaviour."

Jenny says in a petty way, "Fine, I don't like none of you anyway." As she walks off in a sulk.

Russell whispered to Terry, "Psst.... Terry, what's going on with Jenny?" He replied, "She just has a bad attitude. She has always been jealous of me for whatever reason. I think it may be because I am positive and sweet, and she is so bitter, literally."

Mrs Jacket Potato interrupts them, "Can we all please be quiet? I need to introduce you to our new teacher, Miss Sweetheart." Miss Sweetheart smiled and gave a big bubbly welcome. "Hello pupils!" she said as she also gave a big wave, to everyone.

All the pupils sang in unison, "Welcome, Miss Sweetheart."

"Thank you for the lovely welcome, children. As Mrs Jackie Potato stated today, we will have just one lesson today and allow for you to have a bit of a break time in preparation for tomorrow's busy day and schedule. Jackie will take your class today, and today's class will be an art lesson."

Jackie Potato tells the class, "My husband Edward will be stepping up the security and will be our security guard at the school gates while monitoring the lower levels. I want you all to feel at ease and continue with your education. Don't let anyone distract you in life. Stay focused on what you dream to be. So, in today's class, I would like you all to draw exactly what you would like to be in the future before your expiry date. Draw your dreams," she adds.

They all took out their journals and pens and started doodling. When Granny Smith told the children, "My dream is to be a delicious homemade apple pie, one day. As there is nothing worse than wasted food." The class rejoiced and laughed with one another about her dream.

Granny Smith announced that "I nominate Tina Turnip to keep watch with the binoculars." Tina Turnip accepted this and made her way to the opposite shelf, sliding down the garden hose to fetch the binoculars.

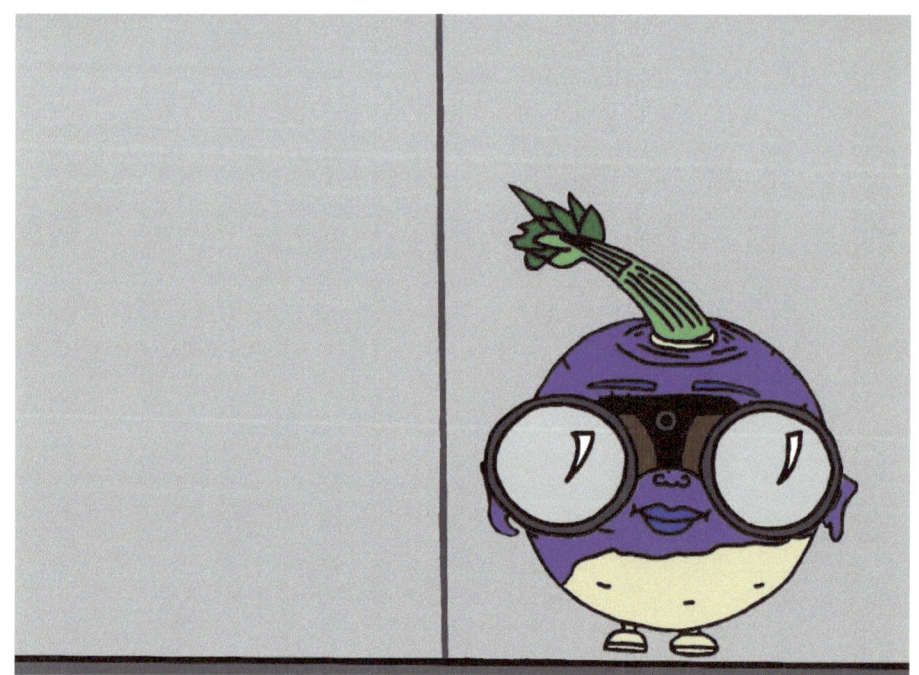

She then retrieved them and made her way back up the garden hose to the highest shelf and started watching what was going on with the other building.

"Miss, before you leave the class, can you tell me what your dream would be before your expiry date," Cherie Tomato asked Miss Sweetheart.

"Yes, of course, Cherie. My dream that I always dreamt about is to be paired up with sausages and mashed potato with lashings of tasty gravy. Yum!" she said while smiling.

The class laughed once again as she emphasised the yum part. Tommy Tomato then asked Jackie Potato. "Jackie, what would you, your husband and Miss Scallion like to be?"

Mrs Jackie Potato spilled the beans. "I know, Miss Scallion very well, and I know for a fact that Miss Scallion often talks about her dream of being added to a salad."

"Boring." Belle Pepper added before asking, "What about Edward and yourself?"

"I have always dreamed of being a delicious and creamy potato salad, ever since I was a baby potato. While Edward has always spoken about being a jacket potato with cheesy beans."

The class were laughing so hard as they continued the sketches of their dreams.

Chapter 4 – Revealing their Dreams and Plans for The Future

Mrs Jackie Potato asked the class to form a line, as one by one, the pupils revealed their future plans and dreams about what they wanted to be when they were older. Russell was the first one in the line, and Jackie Potato asked him, "So, Russell, what do you dream of becoming?"

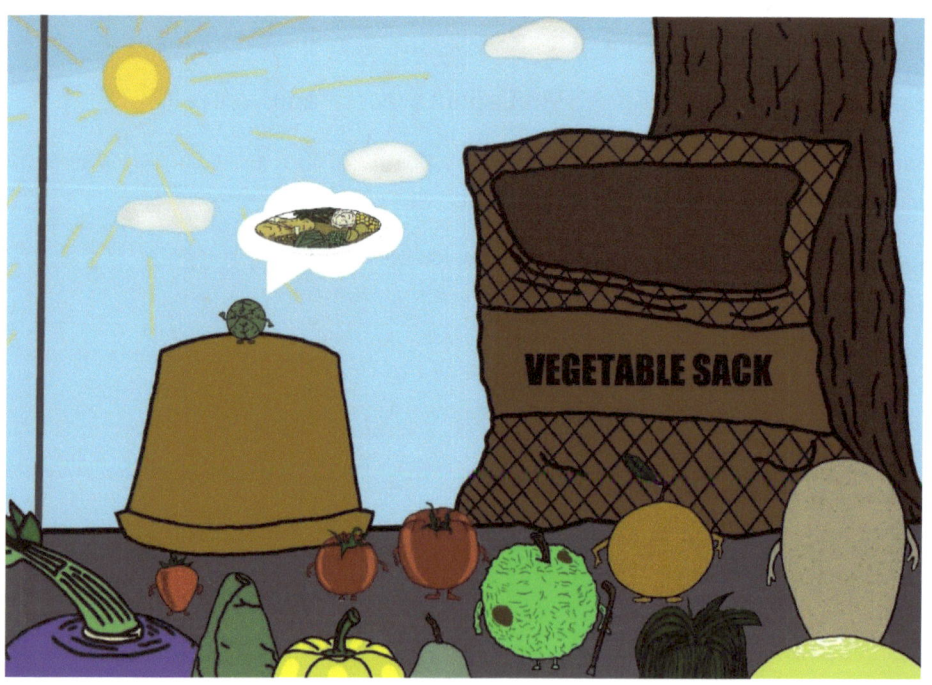

An excited Russell couldn't wait to tell everyone, "I dream one day I will be served up on a plate with other vegetables on a delicious Sunday roast dinner."

"Very, very tasty, Russell—and also very healthy for humans," added Mrs Jackie Potato.

Next in line was Terry Strawberry. He called out, "I would love to be a smoothie, Miss."

Jackie Potato replied to him, "Very sweet, Terry— Ideal for sick humans. Next in line, please."

Jackie looked at Clementine, and without hesitation, she said, "I am happy just to be a snack." Jackie responded, "Never underestimate the importance of healthy snacks—that would be beautiful," she added.

Cherie Tomato spoke up, "I would love to be served on a salad with Miss Scallion." Jackie smiled, nodded and said: "Wonderful, Cherie. A salad can be served with many delicious recipes, a good choice."

Tommy Tomato was annoyed with himself because he was indecisive about what he wanted to be. Then he shouted out, "I am a little uncertain, Miss, as I dream of being two things. I either want to be a tomato soup or a bruschetta—scrummy tomatoes on toast with garlic and basil."

Jackie Potato replied, "Yummy, Tommy—decisions, decisions. Both are incredibly healthy and would benefit any human that is lucky enough to taste them."

Jackie asked. Next in the line, "Cher, what do you dream of becoming?" Cher the pear said, "I am not copying Clem, Miss, but I just want to be a healthy snack. I think it is nice that we are portable and can be eaten or taken anywhere." Jackie responded, "Cher, that is superb. Well done."

Jackie looked at Belle Pepper and asked, "So, Belle, what would you like to be?" Belle Pepper stood firm and proud and replied, "I want to be wrapped in delicious spices with a little bit of a kick. I really want to be inside chicken fajitas."

The class started laughing again, and everyone was enjoying one another's dreams. Mrs Jackie Potato responded, "Belle, you will be mouth-watering for sure."

"Julienne, what would you like to be?" asked Jackie. The carrot flicked her green hair back and said: "I want to be carrot and coriander soup." Jackie replied: "Brilliant! You know soup is very nutritious and healthy."

"Helen Melon, what would you like to be?" asked Jackie Potato. Helen replied, "Well, Miss, my dream is not to be a dish but more of a snack—divided up and kept in the fridge so I can be consumed over a few days." Jackie replied, "Very creative—and why not? That way, you are giving humans one of their five a day over a few days. Very smart."

Jackie called Tina Turnip, who was keeping watch with her binoculars, and asked loudly, "Tina Turnip, what is your dream? What would you like to be when you are older?"

Tina shouted back, "I dream of being a fluffy carrot and turnip mash on a delicious roast dinner." Mrs Jackie Potato shouted back, "Delicious and healthy! You and Russell share the same dream —and hopefully plate."

Julienne the carrot spoke up, "I suppose I wouldn't mind being part of that dream too, but I do dream of being soup more so…" Jackie replied, "Not every carrot needs to be plated up on a roast dinner. As fruit and vegetables, we are all very versatile with a bit of imagination."

Just as the lesson was about to finish Miss Scallion brought back Jenny the Berry from detention. Jenny gave Terry, her brother, another dirty look as the class all looked confused as to why she behaved the way she did.

Jackie Potato said to Jenny, "I hope you'll now behave and that you've learnt your lesson." She followed up with, "Now, what would you like to be, Jenny, when you grow up?"

Jenny the Berry still displayed an attitude problem; she had to be different when she said something that shocked everyone in class, including the teachers. "I don't want to be anything." Jackie responded, "You don't want to make humans healthier? But that is our purpose, our calling. We've been keeping humans healthy since time began. Why would you want to be different?"

Jenny made another ludicrous remark, "I don't care about humans; I don't care about fruit and vegetables either."

Her brother Terry spoke up, "That's because you're selfish and greedy and only care about yourself."

"Shut up. You think you know everything? You think you're better than everyone else?" she responded. The whole class looked at her like she was a spoiled brat. They all shook their heads in disbelief due to her bizarre ranting.

Her brother cannot understand why Jenny is so hateful and angry all the time, but he thinks it's because she doesn't like who she is. Potentially, she has done many things that get under her own skin, but she projects it all onto him because he's positive and everyone else is, and she likes to bring everyone down just because she is unhappy with her choices and actions.

Cher the Pear said to Jenny, "The teachers and the school are trying to help you."

Jenny tells her, "Shut up. Be quiet. No one asked you, Cher."

Miss Scallion lowered herself and bent down to Jenny's level. "I am not sure why you have to act out all the time—but you need to improve your attitude, missy. You are supposed to be sweet, yet you appear very bitter and sour. You don't want to help humans become healthier? Then you'll only become rotten. Is that what you want?"

"I hate this school and all of you. I'll embrace being rotten," Jenny replied. When Miss Scallion said, "Well, you are going about it all the wrong way. If you don't start to behave, you might just find yourself being rotten—and expelled from this school."

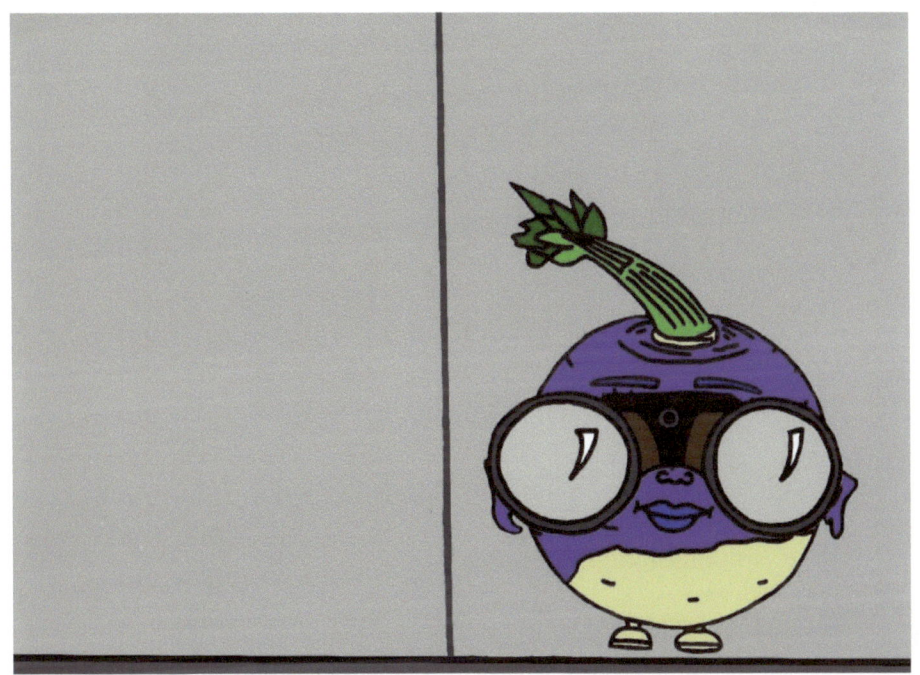

Just as Miss Scallion finished scolding Jenny, Tina Turnip shouted, "I spot something! Three things are making their way towards the school!"

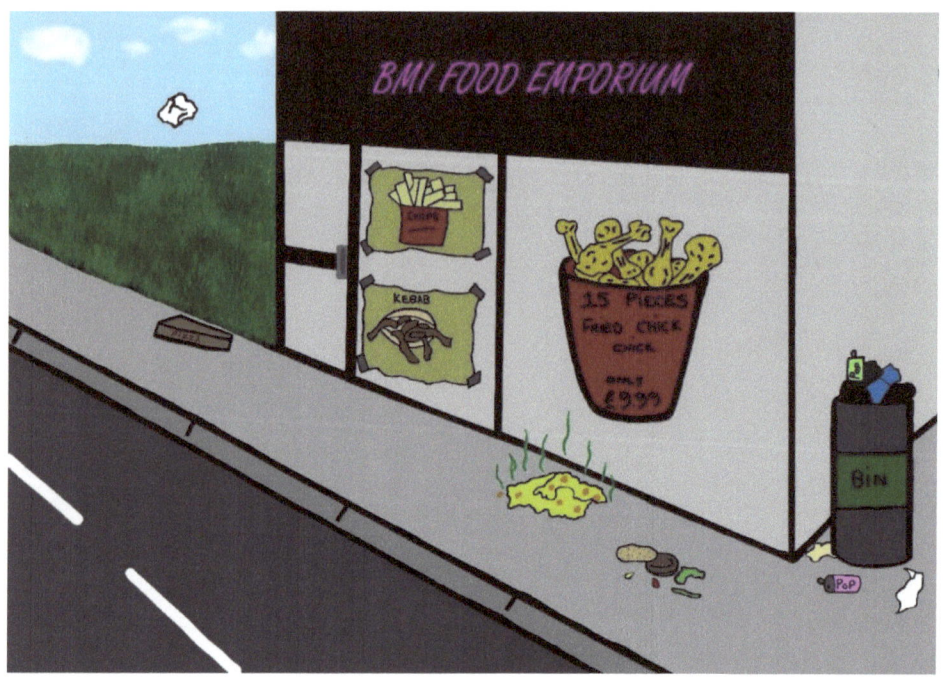

 "What things?" Miss Scallion shouted back. Tina Turnip shouted back again, "I am not sure what they are. I have never seen anything like them before!"

"Class dismissed," said Miss Scallion. "Take a break, children, and we will notify you of your lessons when you return," Jackie Potato added.

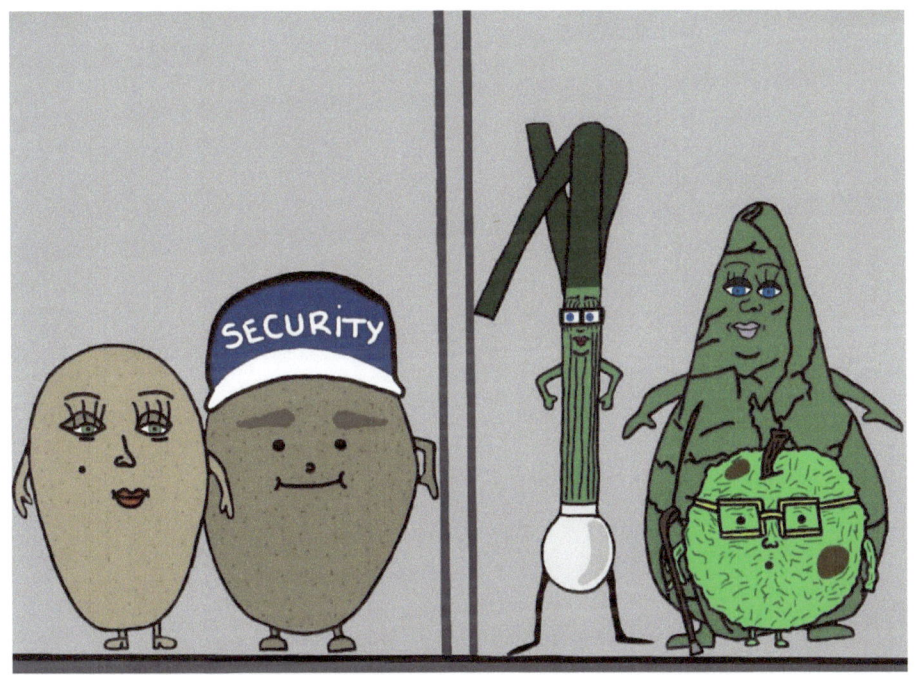

The teachers make their way down to the lower level and report to security Edward Potato. They await the arrival of these three things that are making their way to the school grounds. The fruit and vegetables go and join up with Tina turnip to find out what's going on.

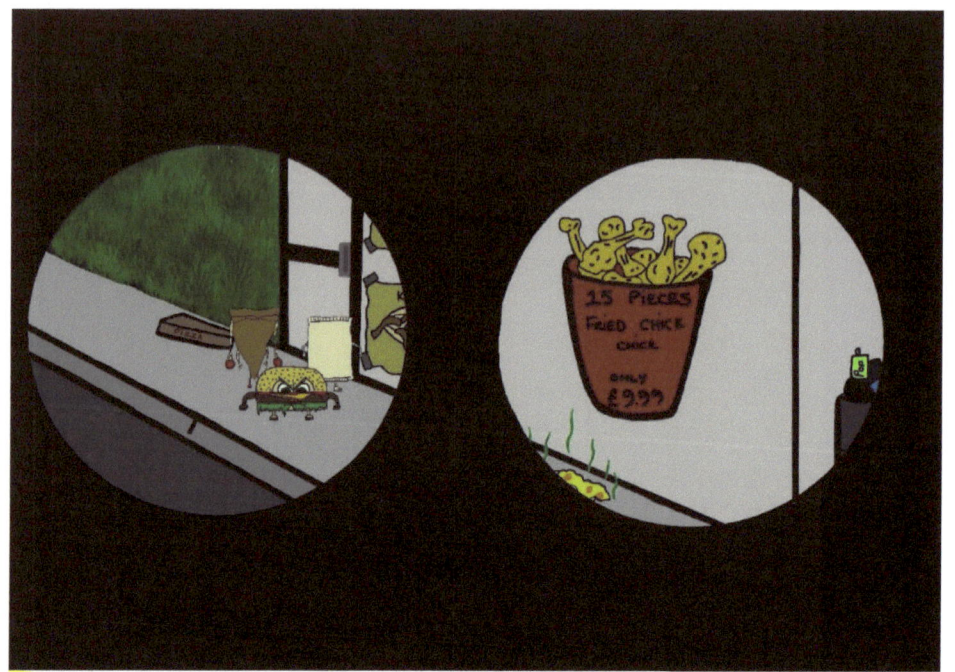

"What can you see?" asked Cherie Tomato. Tina Turnip replied, "I am not sure what they are—but they look gross." Tommy then asked, "Are they definitely coming here?" Tina Turnip responded, "Yes. They will be arriving soon." The class is worrying and doesn't want there day to be ruined. The only one who is happy about the new arrivals is Jenny Berry. The class began to think she had sinister plans or motives.

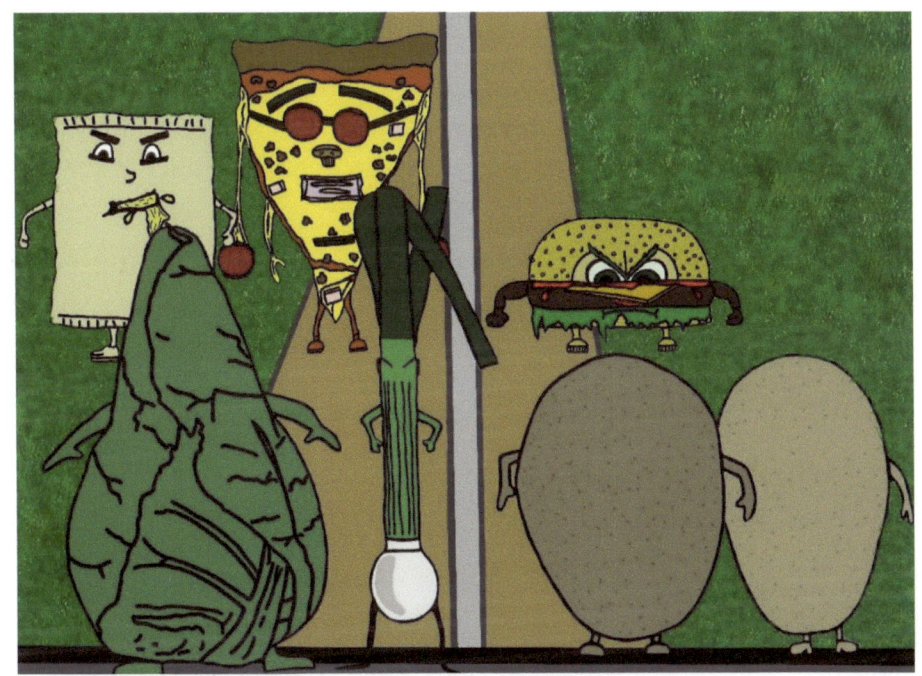

There was a knock on the greenhouse door. The security guard, Edward Potato, Miss Scallion and the other teachers worked together to open the greenhouse door, as they all looked at the new arrivals and were shocked. When Miss Scallion put her hand on Edward's shoulder and said, "I will handle this. Can I help you at all?" she asked, eyeing the strange individuals.

"Hello, can we come in, please?" the odd characters said. Miss Scallion asked them, "Why are you here? What is it that you want?"

The three characters told the vegetables, "The takeaway is shut for the day, and we heard this is a school for food. We have nowhere to go." Miss Scallion was unsure to begin with but felt sorry for the new arrivals and didn't want them to feel unsafe in the outside world.

"The rules here apply to all three of you. You will behave and treat our other pupils with friendship and respect. Otherwise, we will have no other option but to expel you. Today's lessons are English and Biology—so get ready for your lessons." She welcomed them inside. The teachers worked together again to seal the greenhouse door shut.

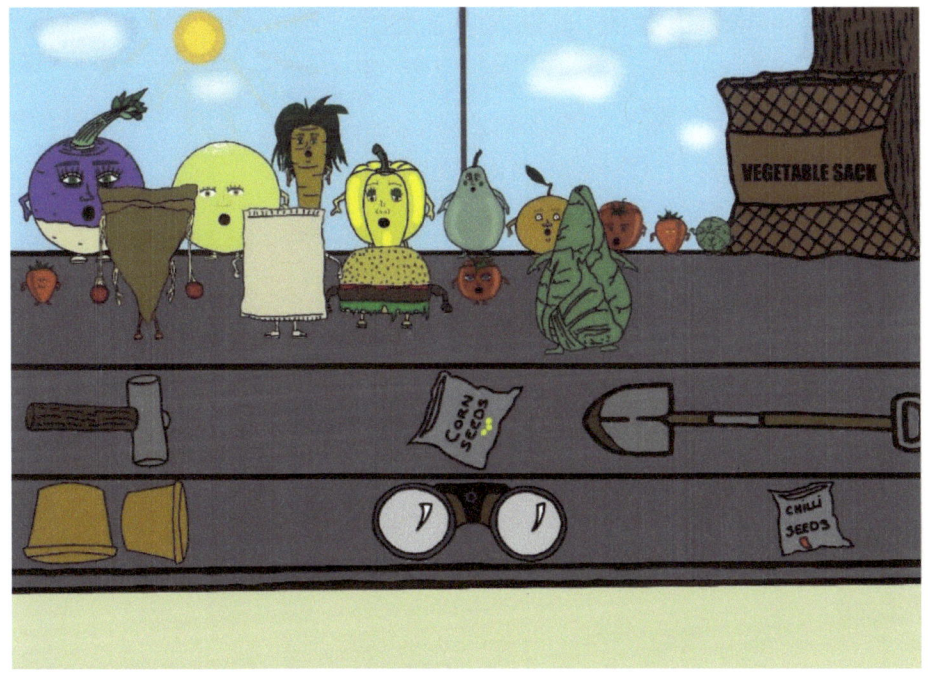

Miss Sweetheart escorted the new pupils to meet the fruit and vegetable pupils. As they made it to the top shelf, all the fruit and vegetable characters looked shocked at the new arrivals. Miss Sweetheart introduced the new pupils to the class. "Excuse me, what are your names?"

"I am Angry Mac," said the burger. "I am Horrid Peter Pizza," added the next. I am Nasty Patsy the Pasty," said the last. Miss Sweetheart replied, "What peculiar names. I hope you can all get along." She walked away to let them get to know one another.

Chapter 5 – Welcoming the New Pupils

The teachers all headed to Miss Scallion's office to discuss the new pupils. As all the teachers were busy, Angry Mac thought he would insert his dominance over the group as all three of the new pupils looked at Russell and ganged up on him.

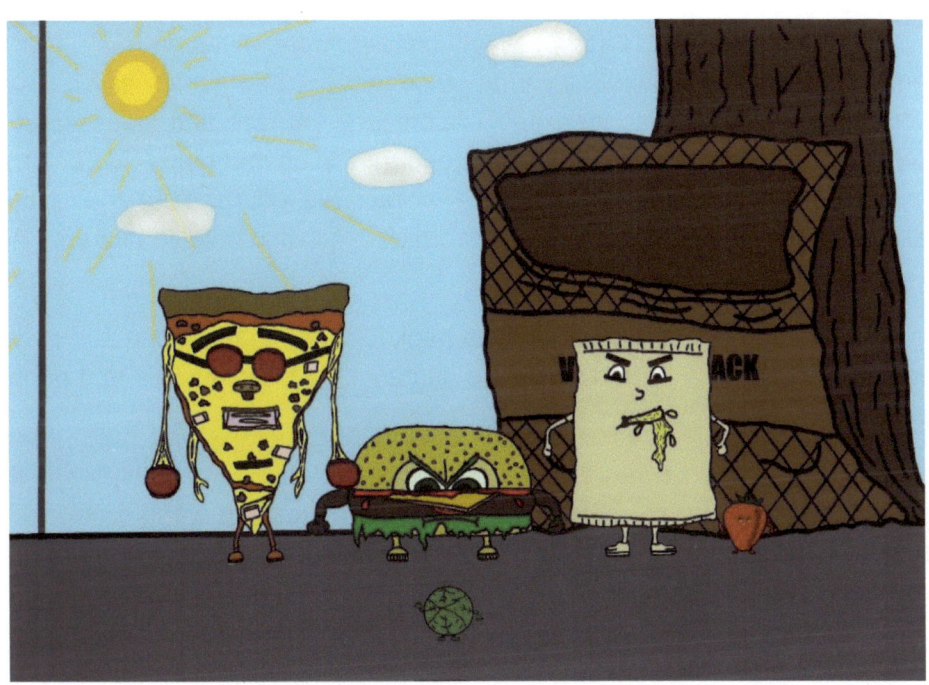

Towering over small Russell, they tried to intimidate and bully him.

"You look just like a bogey," Angry Mac said to Russell as they closed in on him to scare him. Jenny the Berry was the only one out of the class who thought this was funny, as did the bullies. Russell thought he was going to be attacked. When he was saved by the bell, I mean whistle.

All the pupils returned to Miss Scallion and awaited the instruction for the next lesson. "Okay, pupils, it is now time for English with Jackie Potato," said Miss Scallion. Jackie told the class, "It is important to learn English as it helps us communicate better. I would like you all to go to the school library and do some research and study. What we would like you to do is to learn facts about who you are and learn about what makes you special. We are all special in our own rights. We have goodness in us that helps humans; we are packed full of vitamins and minerals that keep humans healthy and strong. This will also give you reasons as to why fruit and vegetables help humans achieve a healthy balanced diet; it will also help you for your next lesson, which is biology," she said.

"Run along now, and when the whistle is blown, come back to us so that we can talk about what you have learned," she added. The pupils all walk in a single file as they take their journals and pens.

They all arrive at the library and start researching themselves. Everyone had their heads down studying when Jenny Berry thought it would be fun to team up with the bullies, she whispers in Angry Mac ear to create havoc for others. She whispered, "Go and give Tommy Tomato a wedgie. Without any care in the world, the three bullies targeted Tommy. Tommy, unaware, was studying when Angry Mac grabbed his skin and, pulled him high off the ground and gave him a wedgie.

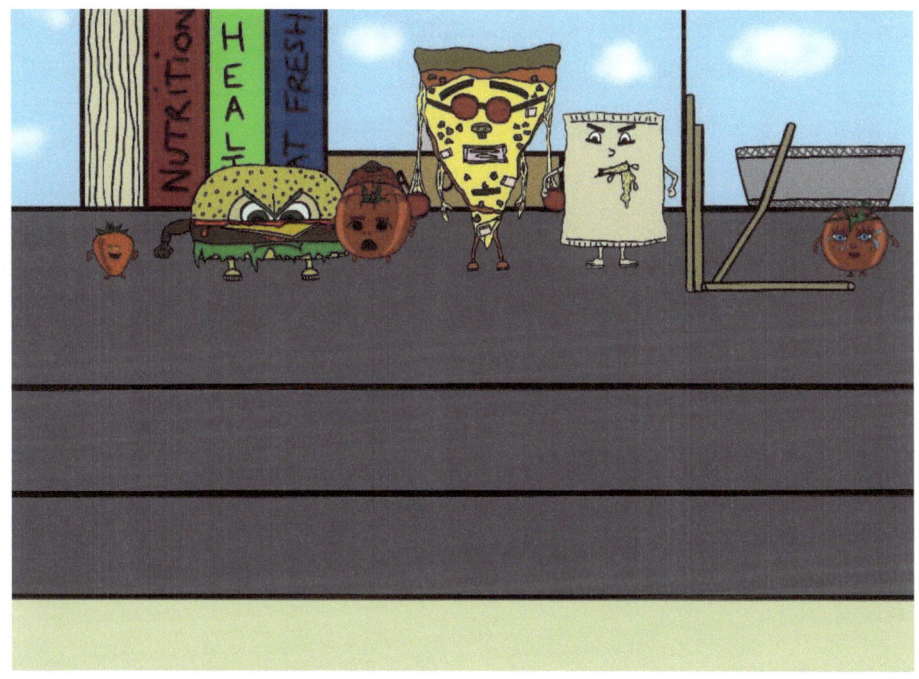

Tommy was calling out, "Ow, put me down. You're stretching my skin." Cherie Tomato looked on in horror and burst into tears. "Please leave Tommy. He is my friend," she begged. Jenny Berry thought it was funny. The whistle was blown, and everyone returned to the teachers and everyone was too scared to say anything in case they were next on the bully chopping board.

Jackie Potato asked the pupils, "Did you do your research? As it will help with your next biology lesson. The pupils answered, "Yes, Miss." Miss Scallion arrived and asked the children, "Did you learn English?"

Clementine spoke, "I learned 'what your name is' in English, Miss Scallion."

"Really, how fascinating what would I be called if I was from the United Kingdom?" she replied. "You would be called Miss Spring onion," Clementine says. The whole class erupt in laughter once more. After reviewing their journals, the teachers realise that the pupils have improved on their writing, there English language and at communicating.

"Class, you have excelled in your English. Well done. It is now time for a break. Have fun and return when you hear the whistle," Miss Scallion said.

Straight away, Jenny Berry was in the ear of Peter Pizza, whispering and being evil, cold and calculated again. Peter Pizza agreed to do what Jenny Berry asked him to do.

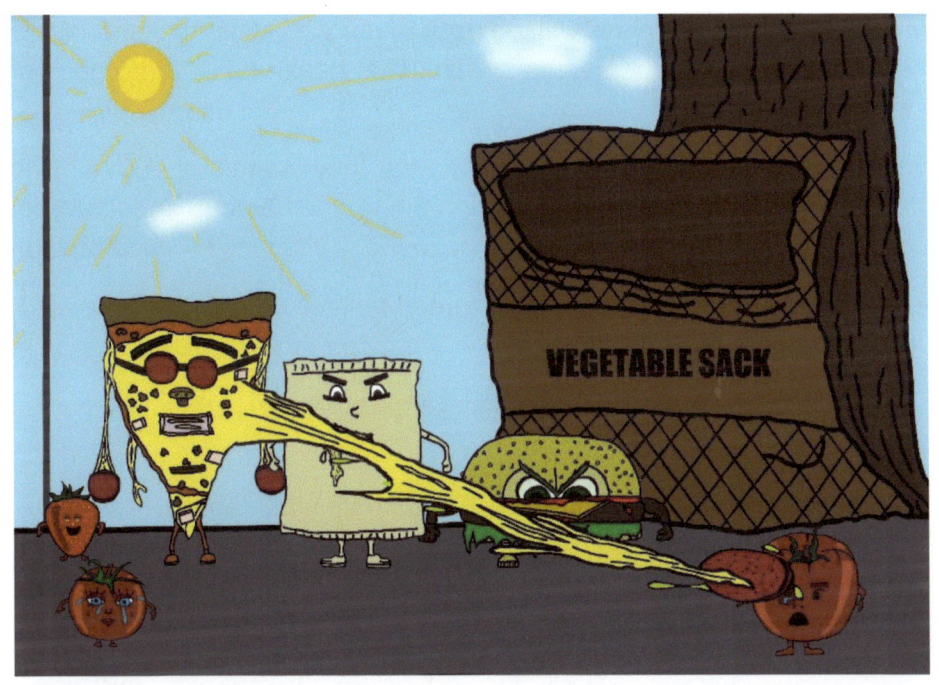

He launched his cheesy pepperoni strands at Tommy's tomato and bruised the skin on his flesh. Cherie cried again. When Miss Sweetheart heard all the commotion, she charged over, "What Is going on here?" she asked. Everyone stayed silent as they feared being targeted next.

Miss Scallion blew her whistle, and the class walked back to her with Miss Sweetheart. "It is time for you all to reveal your superpowers to us in your biology lesson, what health benefits do each of you provide the human with?" she asked as the class got in a single line.

Miss Sweetheart asked, "Everyone in order to disclose what they learned about themselves, starting with Russell." Russell looked at his journal and announced, "I am Russell Sprout, and I have lots of goodness in me. I can improve humans' digestive system, and I contain many vitamins for good health."

The berries are next, and on this rare occasion, they agreed as they both spoke, "We are high in Vitamin C, so a good choice if humans are sick as we support their immune system."

Clementine stood and told the class that I, too, have high levels of vitamin C, which helps reduce inflammation that can cause severe illnesses."

Cher the pear spoke up, "I can help lower cholesterol but improve a human's overall well-being."

Belle Pepper told everyone, "I am high in Vitamin A and C, which can improve skin, hair and nails of humans."

Julienne Carrot told the class, "I have many good vitamins in me, and I can help humans with many things, including strengthening their bones."

Helen Melon spoke: "I have potassium and other vitamins which can help lower blood pressure in humans."

Tina Turnip added, "I help with digestion, I can keep humans fuller for longer and help with blood sugar levels. I just want to point out that all of us have fibre in us, which helps humans lose weight, which means they will be healthier."

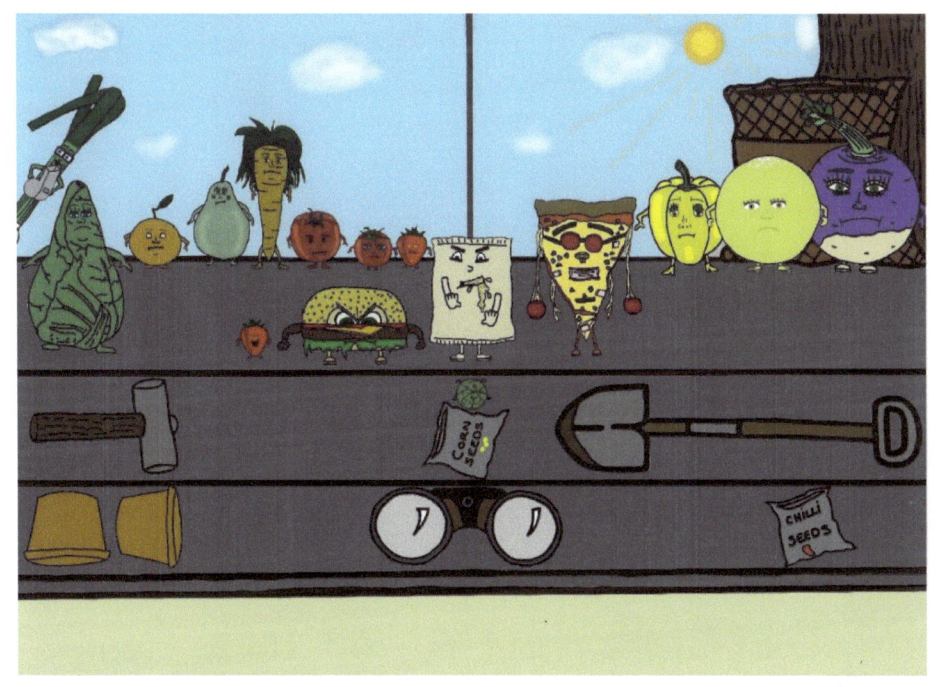

Without warning, the bullies got bored of hearing about all the good qualities of others, and Nasty Patsy Pastry pushed Russell off the shelving in front of everyone as he bounced on the floor below. A furious Miss Scallion had enough. "How dare you push Russell off the shelf? She shouted: "I have no time for bullies. Bullies who team up against one are nothing but weak cowards." Jenny Berry started to laugh, and that was it. Miss Scallion said, "I want you out of my school; Angry Mac, Peter Pizza, Nasty Pasty and Jenny Berry, you are all excluded and must leave the school grounds at once." Miss Sweetheart announced,

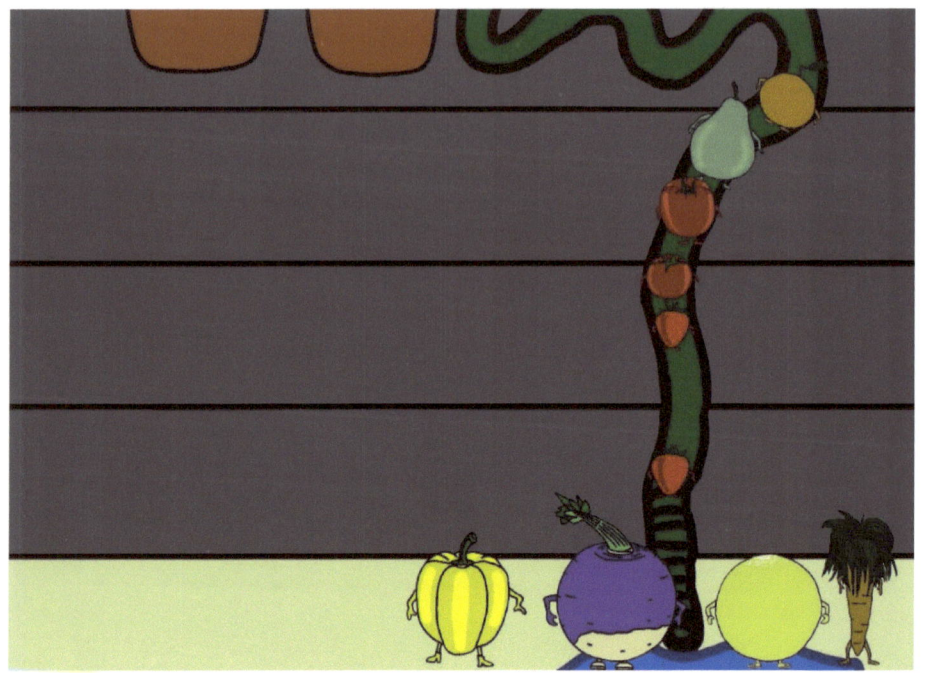

I will escort them off the school grounds," as she walked with all the expelled pupils, they went to the lower levels and saw Russell, who had not even got a mark on him. As Edward Potato, the security guard, took them to the door, Jenny Berry revealed her true colours by pushing Miss Sweetheart through the glass pane. Edward grabbed them all and pushed them out of the greenhouse. Hearing the loud crashing of windows being broken,

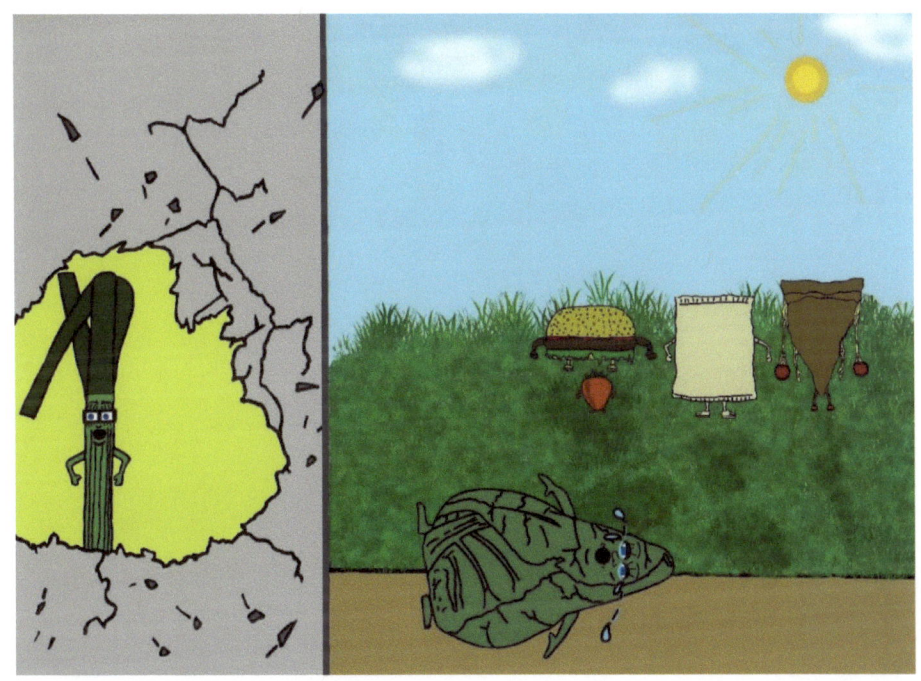

Miss Scallion rushed down to the lower levels of the greenhouse to find poor Miss Sweetheart crying and lying on the floor.

After a terrible day, all pupils headed to the dormitory in disbelief. The teachers arrived and explained everything and tried to make the school a happy school again. They told the fruit and vegetable stories until the moon was back in the sky, and it was time for all students to get some rest.

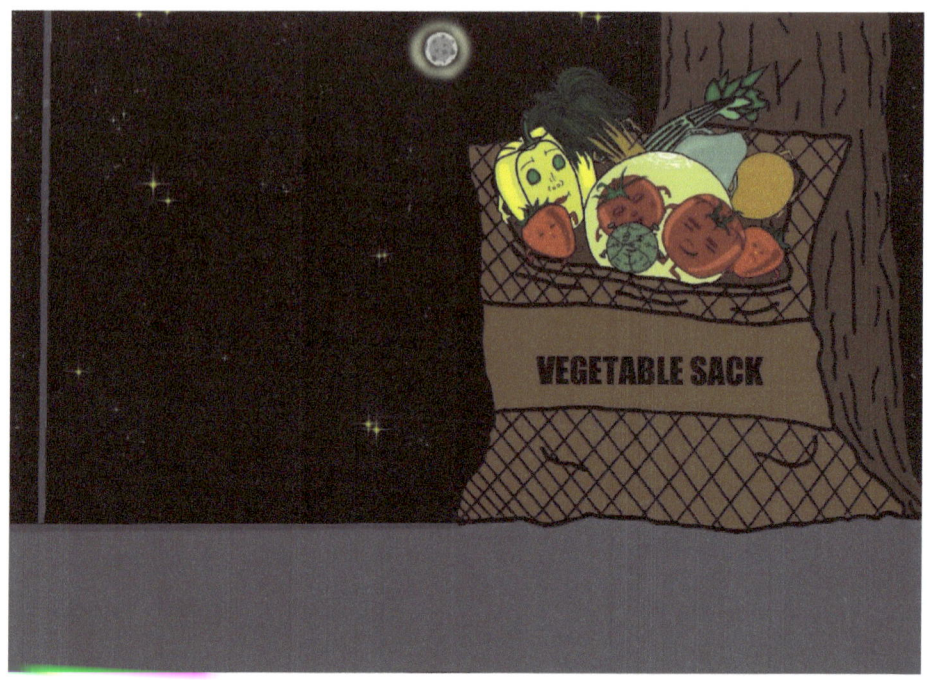

"I wonder what next term will bring," thought Russell before closing his eyes and falling fast asleep.

NHS Guidelines 5 a Day

8 Brussel sprouts is 1

1 medium apple is 1

1 pear is 1

7 Cherry tomatoes is 1

1 slice of Melon is 1

8 spring onions is 1

3 heaped tablespoons spoons of cooked 80g Turnip/Swede is 1

2 clementines is 1

7 strawberries is 1

1 medium size tomato is 1

1 carrot or 3 heaped tablespoons 80g is 1

1/2 a pepper or is 1

80g of mixed vegetable sticks so chopped carrot, peppers, celery etc.

80g of Cabbage/ sweetheart cabbage is 1

Potatoes are carbohydrates which means they don't count as one of your 5 a day, but are still nutritional and contain antioxidants and supply beneficial vitamins and minerals, including vitamin C, B6, and potassium. They may also benefit your digestive health and keep you fuller for longer.

www.ingramcontent.com/pod-product-compliance
Lightning Source LLC
Chambersburg PA
CBHW041116070526
44584CB00002B/188